S

DALY CITY PUBLIC LIBRARY

3 9043 04222471 2

DEC 20 1996

Rough Cuts

D0817076

Daly City Public Library
Daly City, California
DISCARDED

Rough Cuts

A Step-by-Step Guide to
Creating High-Impact Haircuts
. . . at Home!

Roseward Sky

Photographs by Colette Moncíon

Crown Trade Paperbacks

New York

S

646.724
sky

Copyright © 1996 by Crown Publishers, Inc.

All rights reserved. No part of this book may be reproduced or transmitted in any form or by any means, electronic or mechanical, including photocopying, recording, or by any information storage and retrieval system, without permission in writing from the publisher.

Published by Crown Trade Paperbacks, 201 East 50th Street, New York, New York 10022. Member of the Crown Publishing Group.

Random House, Inc. New York, Toronto, London, Sydney, Auckland

http://www.randomhouse.com/

CROWN TRADE PAPERBACKS and colophon are trademarks of Crown Publishers, Inc.

Printed in the United States of America

Library of Congress Cataloging-in-Publication Data is available upon request.

ISBN 0-517-88615-4

10   9   8   7   6   5   4   3   2   1

First Edition

Acknowledgments

This book could not have come to pass without the gracious help of the professionals at salons and schools where hair fashion trends are created:

Learning Institute of Beauty Sciences
New York, New York

New York International Beauty School
Queens, New York

Astor Place Haircutters
New York, New York

The Chop Shop
Brooklyn, New York

Special thanks also to the following people for their support and inspiration:

Genevieve Jones

Lourdes Delda

Juston R. Sky (born 5/24/95—
with a full head of hair)

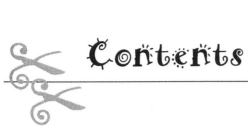

Contents

Rough Cuts

ïntroduction

LET THE WORLD IN ON YOUR ATTITUDE

Not everyone can wear every one, but those who wear them wear them oh-so-well. These cutting-edge styles scream "salon expensive"—but their basically simple designs whisper "you can do it at home!"

They're Rough Cuts, the easy-to-create, hard-to-ignore hair fashions of the '90s.

You've seen Rough Cuts before. Stalking the twilight world of the underground club scene, or blazing a trail in corporate corridors. Signature style of the rising young artist, or finishing touch on the superstar at the Oscars.

Aggressively unique, they're the personal crown of the in-the-know individualist for whom a distinct appearance is a distinct advantage.

Is there a Rough Cut for you? We think so. And can you create it at home in an hour or less? Definitely.

In this book, you'll find some of the coolest cuts going, including savvy asymmetricals, artistic razor cuts, and transgender crop cuts—cuts for every kind of hair. We'll give you step-by-step photos and detailed instructions. From choosing the perfect cut for the shape of your face to using your hair to highlight your best features or make you look (and feel) taller, *Rough Cuts* will help you make the right decisions for you.

Imagine Susan Powter without her trademark crop, Anthony Mason without his razor cut, or Fabio without his flowing mane. A Rough Cut can be the look of your life, or a boost for your lifestyle. Top fashion models know: Wear the right cut and you're on the runway all day, every day.

Ready for takeoff?

GETTING STARTED

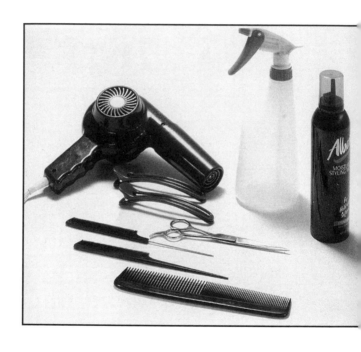

Setting Up

WHERE TO CUT YOUR HAIR

For home hair cutting, you generally have two choices for location: the kitchen or the bathroom. This is where you'll find, all in one place, light, water, outlets, privacy, and surfaces that lend themselves to easy cleanup.

Unfortunately, you usually won't find much operating room in kitchens and bathrooms—so take pains to get rid of clutter before you begin. You'll need lots of room to maneuver.

Also remember to remove shades and covers from lightbulbs to maximize light. Shadows can make your hair look shorter than you intended, and you need maximum light for the best appraisal of your work. Standard, rather than fluorescent, lighting is recommended if you'll be applying color to your hair.

THE TOOLS

Cape

Keeps the hair off your clothes. You can purchase one at any beauty supply store or make one out of a towel or old shirt.

Clippers

Electric clippers (which can only be used on dry hair) are better for creating some of the shorter cuts and for shaping the neckline.

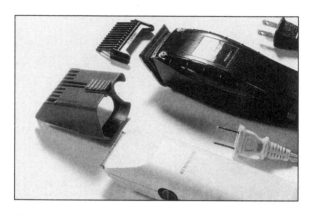

Two types are available: the kind with an adjustable guard and the kind that comes with several guards of different increments of an inch. Adjustable guards tend to slip if you lean on them too hard, so you can accidentally cut your hair too short. Solve this problem by wrapping a thick rubber band around the body of the clipper, which allows the guard to slip no farther back than you want.

With clippers that come with separate, clip-on guards, you risk misplacing the guards, or worse, having one come off the instrument while you're cutting. Bald-spot City. Popular brands are Oster and Wahl. Be sure to read all the instructions that come with the clippers before starting.

Comb

Your comb should lift hair away from the head easily. A large, wide-toothed comb works best for most types of hair. If you have fine hair, try to find a comb that features both wide teeth and finer teeth.

Hair Clips

Clips are necessary for holding sections of hair in place and out of the way. Keep a variety of sizes around for different tasks. Plastic ones are better—they don't rust, and will even stand up to chemicals used in perming and relaxing.

Magic tape

Use as a guideline when you're cutting wet or dry hair. You'll find this fabric tape wherever sewing supplies are sold. Other sorts of adhesive cloth tape will also do, and masking tape's okay in a pinch.

Mirror

We'll assume that your bathroom is equipped with a mirror. If you're not cutting there, you'll need to set up a sturdy mirror wherever you choose to cut. You'll also need a hand-held mirror to view work at the back, sides, and top of your head.

Scissors

A minimum of two pairs of good scissors are necessary: one long-bladed (5½ inches will do), and one short-bladed (3 or 4 inches). The short blades are for precision work, the longer ones for bulk cutting. Quality scissors (price *does* matter) work better than cheap ones, and professional barber shears work best of all.

If all your scissors have sharp points, it may be worth it to invest in a pair with rounded tips. They're less of a safety hazard. Scissors with narrower blades allow you to see the hair more clearly as you cut it.

Test a few pairs, if you can, at your local beauty supply store. They should fit your hand well and feel natural to wield. Revlon makes a good scissor that is available everywhere.

Good scissors can mean the difference between precision and frustration when you cut. Once you have a good pair, never use them on anything but hair, and keep them clean by wiping them off after each cut.

Spray Bottle

Wet hair is more controllable than dry. A spray bottle kept filled with water at hand keeps the hair uniformly wet as you cut.

Styling Brush

A wide-toothed, plastic brush is good for detangling longer hair.

Cutting Basics

The following preliminary steps are required for getting started. Remember, a good start will make for a great finish, so never be tempted to skip the basics.

1. Get to know your hair before you begin to cut. Check in the mirror for any thinning areas, texture changes, cowlicks, or other problems. Straight hair may slick out when it is short, and may require extra length in order to lay down. Cowlicks also need this extra length for better manageability. Take note of such areas on your head and work on them with extra care.

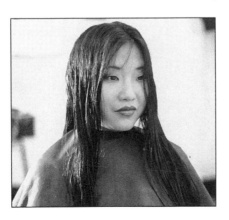

2. Wash, condition, and detangle the hair. Hair that's clean and conditioned is more manageable. Even cuts that will be done dry, using electric clippers, require clean hair in its best condition. Pat the hair dry—hair that's to be cut wet should never be *dripping* wet. Detangle with a wide-toothed plastic brush or comb.

3. Section your hair. Basic sectioning divides the hair into four quadrants, with a part running down the center of the head from back to front, and one running down the horizontal center from right to left. Note which kind of sectioning is required for the cut you desire. Precise sectioning will make for a better haircut.

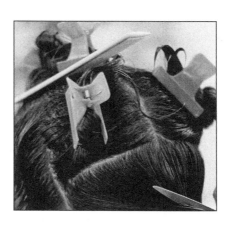

Essential Techniques

Most cuts involve only a few basic techniques.

1. Cut conservatively. Slow, light, cautious cutting, with constant assessment and reassessment of your work, is best. With a conservative approach, you can always cut more if you see fit—but you'll have to live with and regrow hair that's been cut too short.

2. Hair dries shorter than you've cut it while it is wet—especially curly hair. Take that into consideration and cut your hair half an inch to an inch longer than you want it to wind up.

3. Keep an even, steady posture while your hair is being cut. If you sit really still, there's less chance for slipups.

4. Read instructions through and through before embarking on your cut. Familiarity with the steps will prevent misinterpretation.

5. Remember that the crown is the top of your head, the nape is the back of your neck, and the hairline is the edge of hair around your face.

HOLDING HAIR FOR CUTTING

While your dominant hand handles the tools (right if you're right-handed, left if you're left-handed), your other hand handles the hair. Grasp hair for cutting between your index and second finger. Hair, when wet and combed through, should lie between these fingers like a ribbon, making it easy to lift and cut with precision.

With hair in this position, your fingers also act as a cutting guide. To steady your holding hand, always rest it on the scalp (or shoulder for longer hair) as you cut.

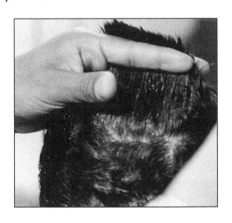

ESTABLISHING GUIDE LENGTHS

For most cuts, you'll have to establish what's known as a guide length, or guideline, to the hair, which you'll use to help measure the rest of the hair you cut. Measure this guide length carefully, as it will determine other lengths around the head. Hold hair with fingers and cut hair above the guide length as shown at left. When we speak of a 2-inch guide length, we mean 2 inches from the scalp. Also, you can use magic tape to hold the hair in place while you cut. Lay tape over the hair at the desired guide length and cut.

When cutting a guide length at the nape of the neck, hold hair straight down along the neck. For a guide length at the crown or at the front of the head, hold hair straight up and away from the head.

RIBBONS AND PIES

A strip of wet hair combed through resembles a ribbon. For convenience, and to help you envision the techniques presented, the instructions often refer to strips of wet hair as ribbons.

Similarly, the term "pie-slice sections of hair" should help you envision sections where parts in the hair meet to create a sort of triangular section of hair. The point of the triangle is the center of the head and the sides move toward the hairline.

LAYERING

Layering, a technique that's part of many cuts, involves cutting many sections of hair in accordance with different preset guide lengths. The main guide is typically established at the crown of the head. You do this by holding a section at the crown straight away from the head (at a 90-degree angle from its base) and cutting it to the length warranted by the haircut you're creating.

When you cut the layered sections beneath it, you'll hold all those sections up to match the length of your guide, and cut. Of course, when the hair lays back onto the head, the ends overlap. Each layer is lower than the next, like shingles on a roof.

FEATHERING

Feathering is a technique used to soften the line of a bang or, to a lesser extent, to blend the edge of a layer in layered styles. Hold your smaller scissors at almost a right angle to the line you're cutting into the hair and lightly snip nicks into the ends of the hairs.

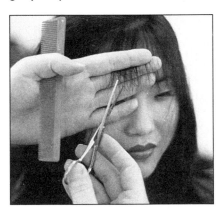

Now you're ready to choose a cut!

THE CUTS

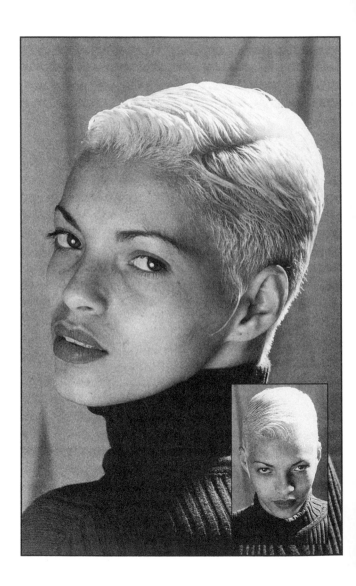

Platinum Butta

Here's where easy care takes on an edge. This short creation is reminiscent of the Caesar style popular among men, and every bit as assertive when teamed up with female beauty. The steps involved require both scissor and clipper work. Therefore, the cut must be done while the hair is dry.

Cropped, bleached, and colored for dramatic effect, Dorothy's naturally black hair will need to be touched up frequently (with permanent color) to maintain the look. But it fits her so well that it's worth it! Her oval-shaped face is suited for almost any cut, and this one shows off her best features in an eye-catching way.

The cut is longer at the crown than at the sides, with a thin tendril left long over each ear.

🕐 60 minutes

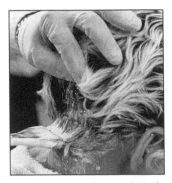

Step 1•Section hair and apply bleach starting at nape of neck.

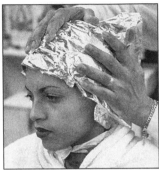

Step 2•Work bleach into hair for even coverage. Leave bleach on for about 30 minutes. Rinse thoroughly and dry. (This short creation requires scissor and clipper work. Therefore, the hair is cut dry.)

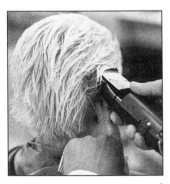

Step 3•Using a generous guard on clippers, cut upward from the nape of the neck and from the earline toward the crown.

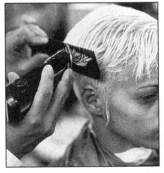

Step 4•Use the comb to lift the hair. Keep electric clippers underneath the comb. Leave a long tendril at each sideburn, an important feminizing detail.

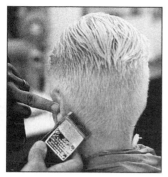

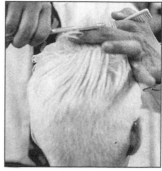

Step 5•Taper the sides and back downward using a ¼-inch guard. Cut up and away from the head in short arching motions. Leave hair about ¾ inch long just below the crown.

Step 6•Create a layered bang. Comb hair forward from about ½ inch behind the hairline. Establish a 2-inch guideline at the center and outer sides of bang. Connect guidelines with a gentle curved line.

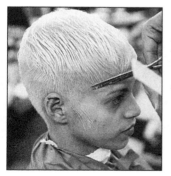

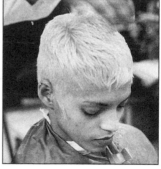

Step 7•Comb forward, then cut a second section of hair behind the bang according to the length of the original guideline. Repeat this step until you can no longer pull hair toward the guideline for the bang.

Step 8•Comb and style.

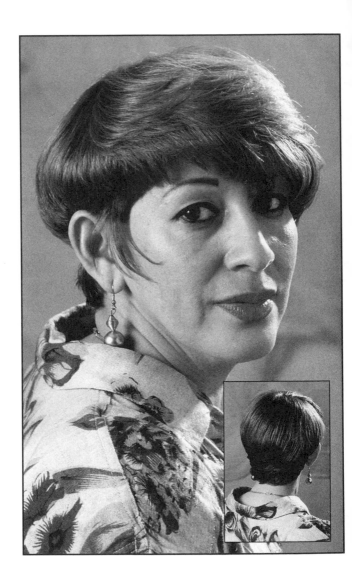

Seventh Avenue

For women who want an easy-care cut, but are cautious about going too short, the asymmetrical Seventh Avenue is a cut to consider. It leaves enough fullness on top and offers enough movement to show off the hair, yet retains the chic lines and simplicity of a short cut.

Roslyn's hair is full and healthy looking, but her original short, layered cut didn't show it off to its best advantage. The Seventh Avenue complements her oval face and open features.

The Seventh Avenue leaves volume at the crown, and long accents at the ear. The rest is cut short in an underlayer, giving the cut sleek lines and a high-fashion look.

🕐 45 minutes

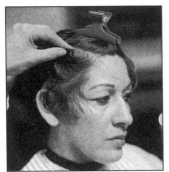

Step 1•While wet, section top and sides of hair. Create a 4-inch perimeter guide length at the earline on the right side. Leave a layer of tendrils beneath the guide length. Tendrils are an essential detail.

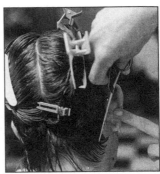

Step 2•Working on the right side of the head, bring ribbons of hair from the crown to meet the perimeter guide length and cut.

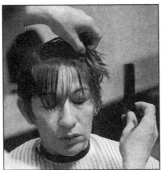

Step 3•On the left side of head, establish a 5-inch guide length. The two lengths will blend together in the back of the head. Remember, this is an asymmetrical cut and the hair should be longer on the left.

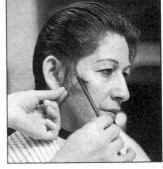

Step 4•You've now cut all the hair below the perimeter to match the guide lengths. Next, comb all the hair straight down in preparation for creating the uppermost layer of hair and the bang.

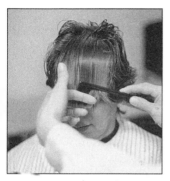

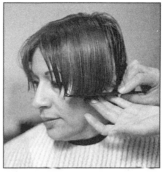

Step 5•Cut guide length 7 to 9-inches long, depending on how long you'd like the uppermost layer of hair to be when dry. Draw ribbons from rear of the crown working your way left. Cut to match guide length.

Step 6•Hair will hang in a blunt layer just below the cheekbone. Trim the rear line of this layer to merge smoothly from the shorter hair on the right side of the head to the longer hair on the left.

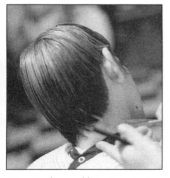

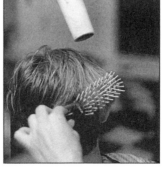

Step 7•The neckline is cut at a stylish angle using the comb as a guide.

Step 8•Dry and style.

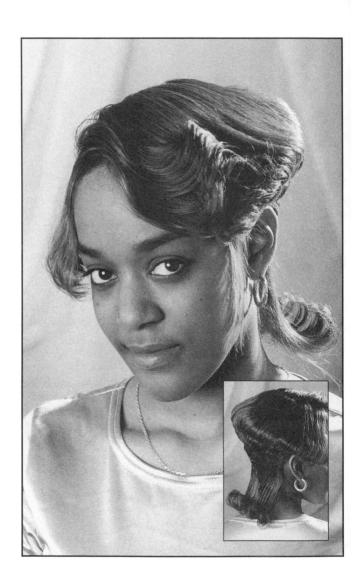

Petals

A Petals cut puts the hair on display. Layered in the back, with length along the neck and curled or flipped on top, this cut also shows off color well. And it's surprisingly simple to create.

The Petals cut makes use of the electric clipper, and should be done dry. Lora's hair was already layered and sheared to a taper at the back. To taper, section off hair between the crown and nape of the neck. Begin bulk-cutting using an electric clipper guard of ½ inch or more. Lift the hair at the sides and back and cut upward at the root. This leaves enough hair at the back and sides to taper later.

The Petals cut has length on top, a side part, accents at the ears, a sharp, layered wedge at the back, and a longer "bang" at the neck.

⏲ 60 minutes

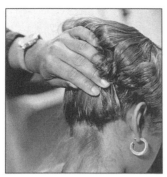

Step 1•Cut the hair dry. Separate a 5-inch length of hair at the nape of the neck.

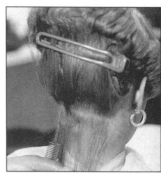

Step 2•Trim the ends, twist, and section off with a clip.

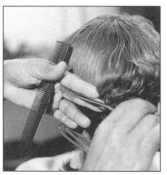

Step 3•Create a mushroom effect at the rear of the crown by establishing a 4-inch guideline at the crown and bringing up horizontal ribbons from all around the crown for cutting.

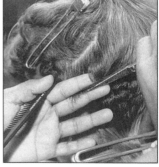

Step 4•Working around the head, blend the longer top sections by grasping vertical ribbons of hair and cutting them along a 45-degree angle. Cut both bangs and back of hair using the fingers as a guide.

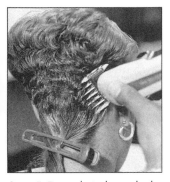

Step 5•Taper hair beneath the mushroom. Cut hair longer immediately beneath with a scissor, and taper lower hair with electric clippers.

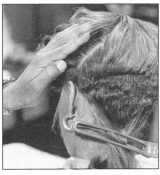

Step 6•Note that hair is tapered in gentle layers.

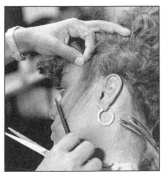

Step 7•Establish a 2½-inch guideline for the tendrils, which are kept long on each side.

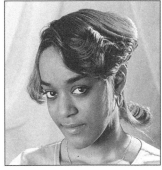

Step 8•Brush top to the side. Curl into a soft bang.

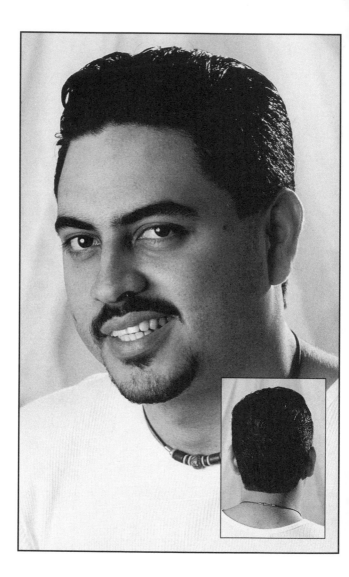

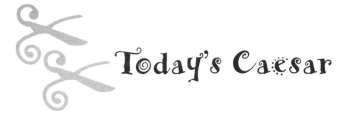

Today's Caesar

It is as easy to create a hot cut for a guy as it is for a gal. Winston's oval face will wear the Caesar cut well, and the rakishness of the style is perfectly accented by his light goatee.

The Caesar is fuller on top than at the sides and can be combed forward or backward for two distinct looks.

🕐 30 minutes

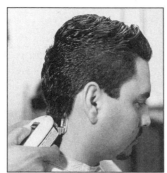

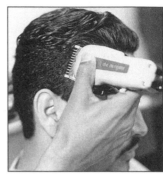

Step 1•Taper dry hair at back and sides using electric clippers.

Step 2•The hair toward the crown should end up about ¾ inch long and be tapered to about ¼ inch long at nape of neck.

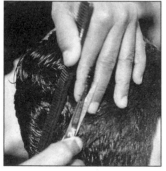

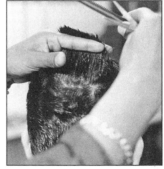

Step 3•The back and sides are blended with longer hair at the crown. Use scissors or electric clippers and comb.

Step 4•The hair at the top of the back of the head is cut to match a 2-inch guideline at the crown.

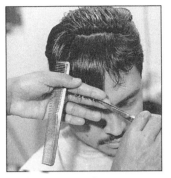

Step 5•Divide the hair on the top of the head into two halves. You'll be turning the front half into a bang.

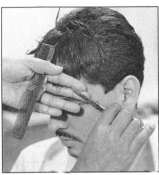

Step 6•Establish a 3-inch guideline for the bang. Note the hairline around the face is shaped with clippers.

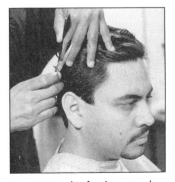

Step 7•Put the finishing touches on the cut. Hold vertical ribbons of hair on an angle. Cut longer toward the top, shorter toward the bottom.

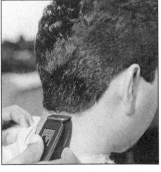

Step 8•Clean up edges with clippers. Gel and style.

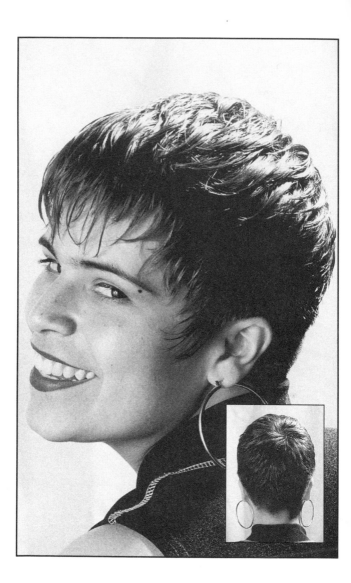

The Tango

Cheerful, feathered, wash-and-go, this eye-emphasizing cut is popping up in the most out-of-the-way "in" spots. The fact that it takes a certain verve to step up to the Tango, however, assures that you won't soon see them on just anyone. Wear yours with that in mind.

Mary started off with very long, full hair. It requires more elaborate sectioning to prepare long hair for cutting. Each section of hair is shortened considerably before the shaping of the style begins.

Despite of the "even all over" look of this cut, it's actually much longer at the crown than it is at the sides and back. Careful tapering of the hair accomplishes the even effect.

🕐 60 minutes

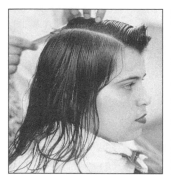

Step 1•Cut the hair wet. If you're starting with long hair, follow steps 2–6 to bulk cut the hair short.

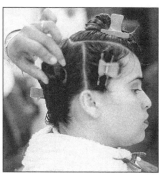

Step 2•To bulk cut, first section the hair with clips.

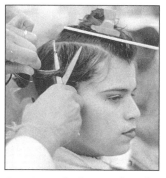

Step 3•Cut the hair on the sides close to the head, leaving about 6–7 inches.

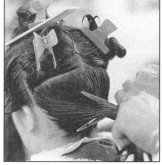

Step 4•Cut the hair in the back to the same length.

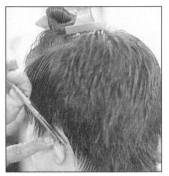

Step 5•Work with scissors to shape hair around the sides.

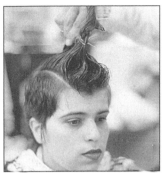

Step 6•Snip the top. Leave about 5 inches, and a 2½-inch tendril at each ear.

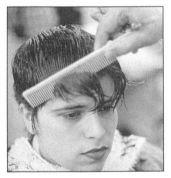

Step 7•Comb all hair forward into a bang. The hair should fall in layers.

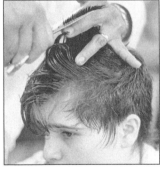

Step 8•Establish a 5-inch guideline for the crown, and cut hair to match.

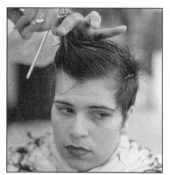

Step 9•Continue to match top layer to guideline.

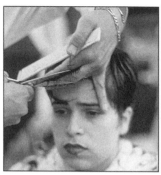

Step 10•Trim bang to just above eyebrows.

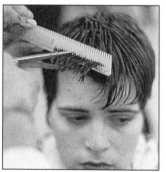

Step 11•Feather the edges.

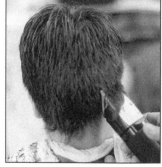

Step 12•Using a ¼-inch guard, taper the back and sides of the hair with electric clippers.

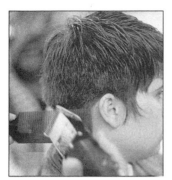

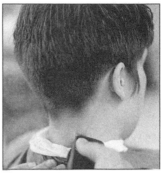

Step 13•Feather tendrils to 2½ inches and adjust hairline at sides and back.

Step 14•Use clippers to blend the hair at sides and rear with longer top section. Clean neckline with clippers.

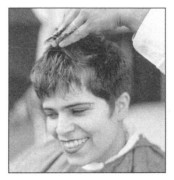

Step 15•Blow dry forward toward face.

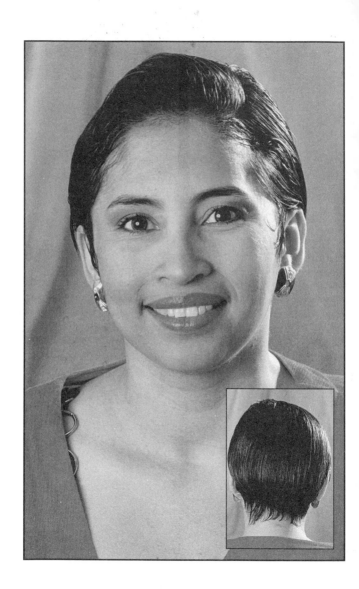

The Flipped Script

The Flipped Script—an easy style that matches the mood of your attire, whatever you're wearing. Dress conservatively and the style is conservatively fashionable. Dress high-fashion and the style is sleek, streamlined, avant-garde. On Jenny, whose classic profile, wide smile, and large eyes perfectly complement the cut, the Flipped Script is a subtle statement that's hard to overlook. You'll be surprised by how simple it is to create.

For The Flipped Script, an underlayer of shorter hair begins at the nape of the neck. Longer hair at the back of the head covers it. At and near the crown, longer hair makes for plenty of volume.

45 minutes

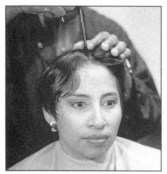

Step 1•Cut the hair dry.

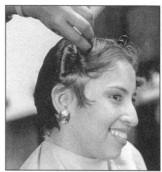

Step 2•Section the hair in front and sides, and separate with clips. Section hair for the sideburn.

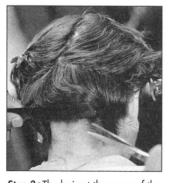

Step 3•The hair at the nape of the neck is cut first. Underlayer of hair at nape is cut in short layers, about 1½ inches.

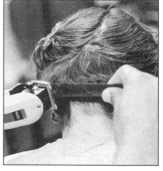

Step 4•Clean up the neckline with electric clippers.

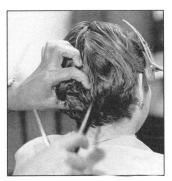

Step 5•Comb hair directly down over the underlayer and cut to about 3 inches long in the center, and about 2½ inches long at each side.

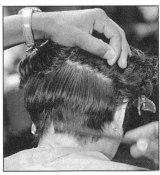

Step 6•Cutting toward the center, connect the sides with the center.

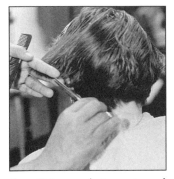

Step 7•Longer hair on top of head, including the bangs, is drawn in vertical ribbons and cut all the way around to match a 6-inch guide.

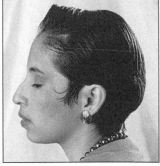

Step 8•Feather the sideburns. Pull part of the bangs over and the rest straight back. Comb and style.

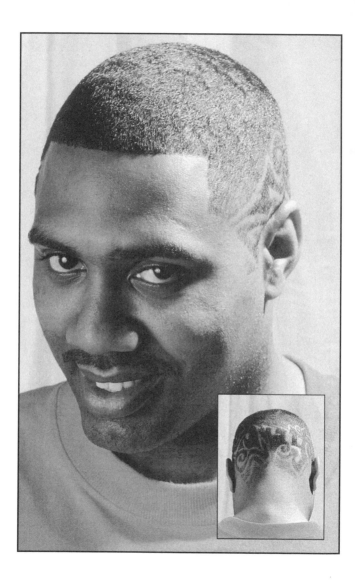

Razor Cuts

Using the corner of an electric clipper, a steady hand, and the human head as your canvas, you can create a masterpiece. Razor Cuts typically adorn the sides and back of the head, and begin to grow out within three or four days. Tips for Razor Cuts:

- Be sure to work with short hair. The longer the hair, the less well-defined your Razor Cut will appear.

- Have an idea for the artwork in mind before you begin. Draw it on paper, and revise it there until you're happy with it. (Once it's been cut into the hair, no revision is possible for a while.)

- Work slowly, with patience. It's easy to mess up a razor cut—and just as easy to complete it without mistakes, if you take the time to do it right.

⏰ 45 minutes

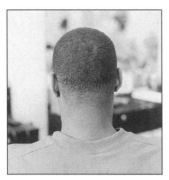

Step 1•Use electric clippers on the hair to achieve an even ¾-inch length all over.

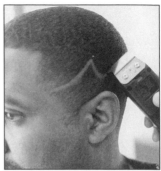

Step 2•Think about the design you want to create: free-form, mountains, landscape, geometric shapes, names, or words.

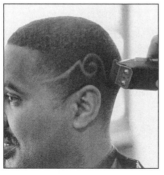

Step 3•Start at the left side and use the edge of the bare clipper to create your design.

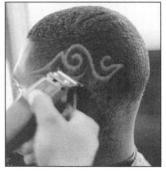

Step 4•Do not rush. Move around the head from left to right.

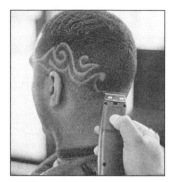

Step 5•Use clippers with a steady hand.

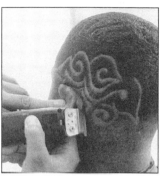

Step 6•Be careful to define the design below the ear.

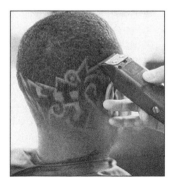

Step 7•Almost done. . . .

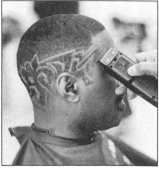

Step 8•The finished product.

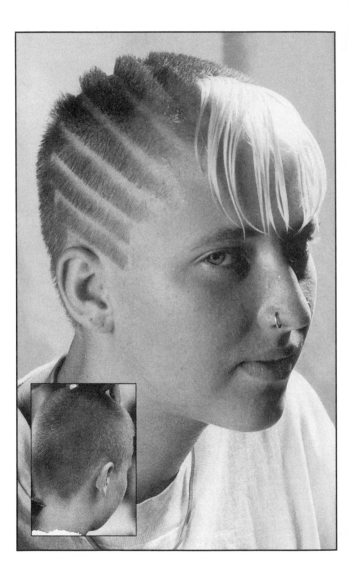

Forelock

You'll turn heads with the Forelock. This razor style has terraces and a bleached, feathered bang. Use the clippers to cut vertical or sloping lines to create a raised effect.

If you wish, you can omit the terraces and leave your hair at stage one, a barely-there shortcut. You can even graduate the hair and ease into the popular Fade, longer on top and disappearing at the nape of the neck.

🕐 45 minutes

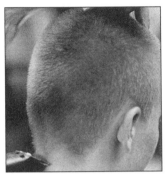

Step 1•Cut the hair while dry. Starting with long hair, simple bulk cutting using an adjustable guide achieves an even ¾-inch length all over, except for the bangs, which you leave 6 inches long.

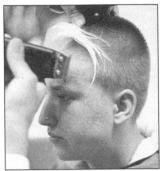

Step 2•Use electric clippers to shape hairline. Note the bang is bleached for contrast.

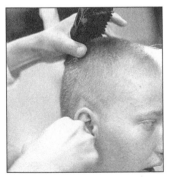

Step 3•The earline is cut to achieve a chic angle just at the top of the ear.

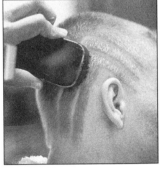

Step 4•Use a brush to remove stray hairs. Use the edge of your bare clipper to cut parallel right angles on one side of the head until you reach the center of the back of the head.

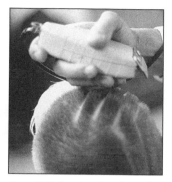

Step 5•Take time to draw the lines.

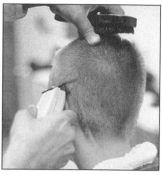

Step 6•Cut terraces on the other side of the head.

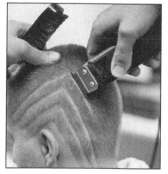

Step 7•Note the symmetry of the lines on both sides.

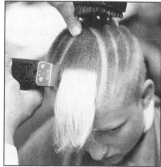

Step 8•Trim the ends of the bangs. What color will you wear them?

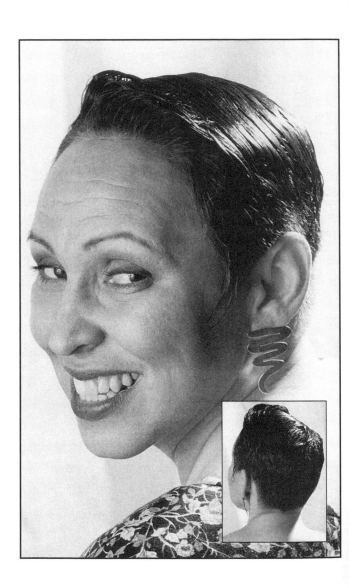

Tangerine

Parted on the side, short in the back, and layered on top, Tangerine is the perfect summer cut. If your hair is curly like Angie's, a light relaxer and gel will straighten it so the longer hair at the crown will lay flat.

If cut even shorter on the sides and back and left long on top, this cut is the Blowout for men. Tangerine is a great transgender look. Wear it with your beach beau!

🕐 40 minutes

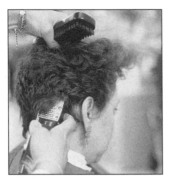

Step 1•Use electric clippers to bulk cut dry hair at the back and sides of the hair up to the crown.

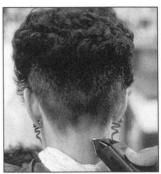

Step 2•Layer the back of the hair so that each layer is about 1½ inches long. Shape the hair at the nape of the neck.

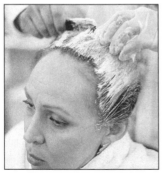

Step 3•Apply a chemical straightener to relax the curl in the hair if desired. Follow the directions on the product you're using. Or, wash the hair and leave wet in preparation for further cutting.

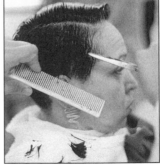

Step 4•Cut a guide length in wet hair at the rear and sides of the crown. The guide should be about 7 inches and will establish the topmost layer of hair, around the head.

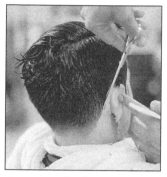

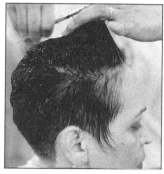

Step 5•Trim hairline at sides with scissors. Leave enough hair by the ears for 2½-inch tendrils.

Step 6•Establish a 5-inch guide length at the front of the crown, and cut. Trim and feather tendrils.

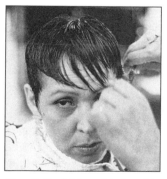

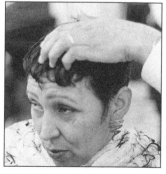

Step 7•Establish a 3-inch guide length for the bangs.

Step 8•Dry and style.

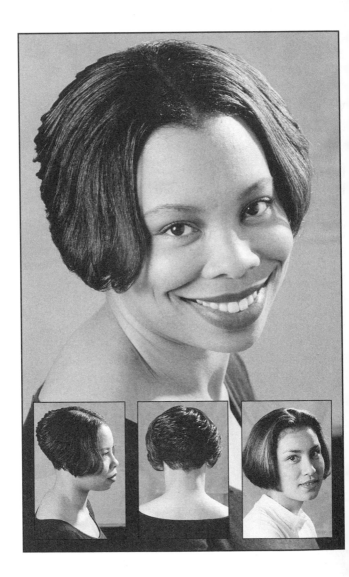

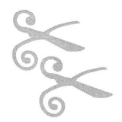

Flashpoint

With its dramatic angle and voluminous layering at the back, the Flashpoint is a perfect cut for high fashion, high cheekbones, and high times. The versatility of the cut is also a plus. Created with similar steps to Petals, the Flashpoint leaves plenty of hair at the crown to experiment with a range of styles. The shorter hair at the nape of the neck is layered and tapered. The longer hair at the crown falls over the tapered hair underneath.

🕐 40 minutes

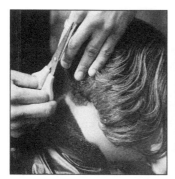

Step 1•Cut the hair while dry. To create the uppermost layer of hair around the crown, establish a guide length at the rear of the crown. Cut to match this guide length of 4–5 inches.

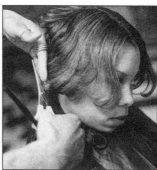

Step 2•Bring hair from the crown, including the front, to match the guide length, and cut.

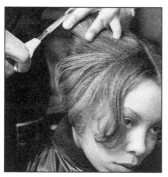

Be careful to follow your guide length.

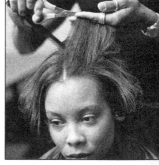

Step 3•As you cut, hair at the sides of the face will naturally end up hanging longer than hair at the back of the head.

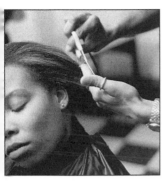

Step 4•Once the upper layer has been cut, section off with a clip. Now you will taper the hair at the neck.

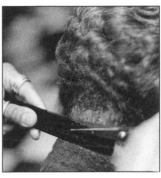

Step 5•Begin bulk cutting hair at the nape of the neck using an electric clipper guard of ½ inch. Lift hair at the sides and back, and cut upward at the root. The hair should be 3 inches long at the rear of the crown and ½ inch at the nape.

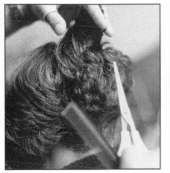

Step 6•Using your fingers as a guide, blend the hair at the tapered section at the back with hair from the uppermost layer.

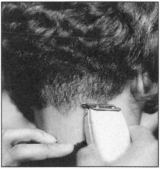

Step 7•Use clippers to shape the neckline into a double U.

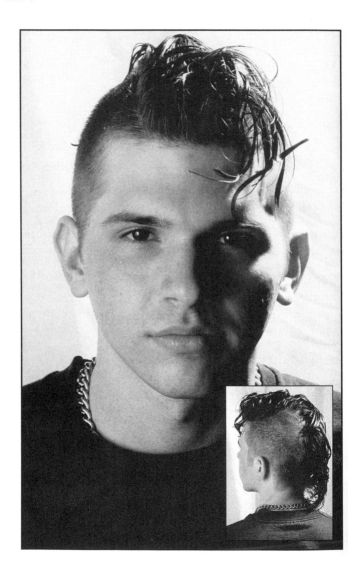

Soho/The Village

Imagine the looks you'd get asking the average barber to give you this cut! Why not make your own statement—literally—with the help of electric clippers, scissors, styling gel, and a few hair clips.

The hair is sheared on the sides to show off the central mane of hair that flows down the middle of the head. Vertical part lines center the mane. This post-punk Mohawk's guaranteed to widen small-town eyes. But then again, that's half the fun of it!

⏱ 40 minutes

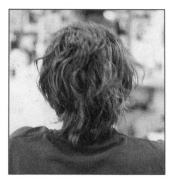

Step 1•Cut the hair while dry to about 6–7 inches all over. Centering the Mohawk on the head is the key to this cut. Comb hair and plan where to position the mane.

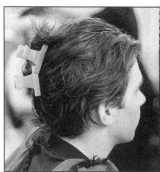

Step 2•Section a 1- to 2-inch-wide strip at the center back. Separate with a clip.

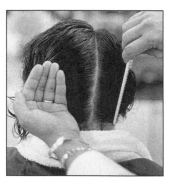

Step 3•Make a vertical part on each side of the center section of the head from the crown to the nape of the neck.

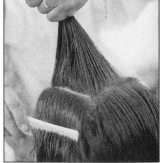

Step 4•Section off the center top and twist. Comb the sides away from the center. Be sure the parts are clean.

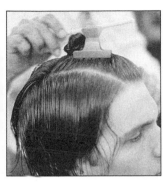

Step 5•Separate top with a clip.

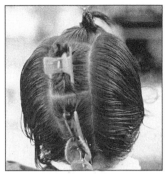

Step 6•Center section is divided and clipped. The width of the mane should narrow very gradually toward the nape of the neck.

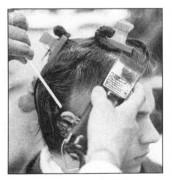

Step 7•Shear the side of the head with electric clippers. Use a guide that allows a ¼ inch of hair or less. Do not cross your center part lines. Shear away from, rather than toward, the part lines.

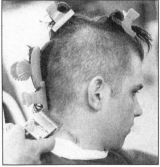

Step 8•Using the bare clippers, create sideburns and shape the hairline.

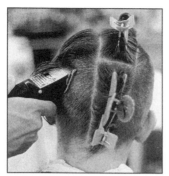

Step 9•Repeat the same steps on the other side. Remember to leave the central mane untouched.

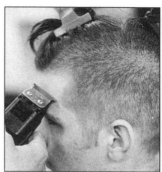

Step 10•A side view. Clean up the hairline with electric clippers.

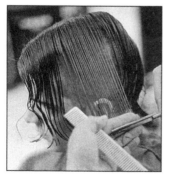

Step 11•Remove the clips from the mane. Comb hair over to one side of the head. Trim the ends with scissors, leaving the hair as long as you can.

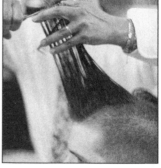

Step 12•Extend ribbon of hair at top of head. Cut to match a 6-inch guideline.

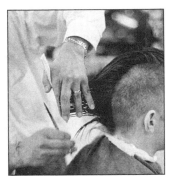

Step 13•Even and trim ends from top of crown to nape of neck.

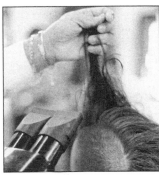

Step 14•Blow out the mane.

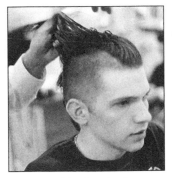

Step 15•Add gel and style.

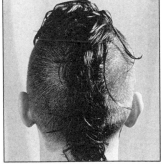

Step 16•Finished back view.

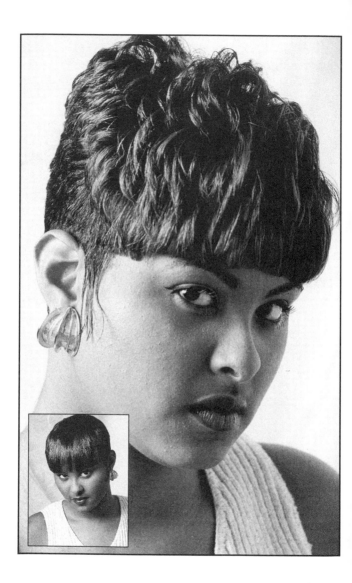

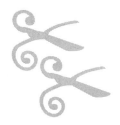

Spun Sugar

Spun Sugar—a cool summer look, is for the more daring. It requires even features and an eye for accessories. Lillian has another asset that's perfect for this cut—a neat, round, head and face.

Surprisingly, the cut is easy to create. Eyebrow length bangs cap the head all the way around to create a mushroom effect. The hair in the back below the mushroom is tapered very short. Note the versatility of the cut shown here: worn straight, its sleek lines are uncompromising and sophisticated. With body-adding waves, the look is softer and more feminine.

🕐 45 minutes

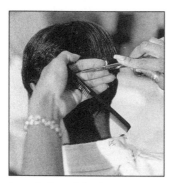

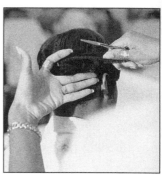

Step 1•Cut while dry. To create the beginning of the mushroom, start at the ear. Divide hair, creating an ear-to-ear part extending across the top of the head. Comb half forward and half back.

Step 2•The half of the hair that is combed back is cut in 5-inch layers using scissors. Taper the hair in the back using directions on page 67.

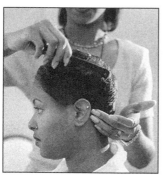

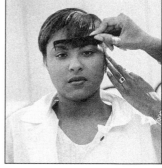

Step 3•Examine the cut to be sure the shape of the mushroom is established before proceeding to the bang. Comb all hair forward to make bang.

Step 4•Establish a 5-inch guideline for the bang. This bang reaches the eyebrows and requires a straight line all the way across.

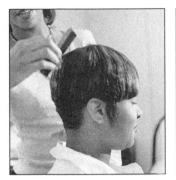

Step 5•Comb hair into place. Trim sides of the mushroom to blend with the bang. Do not cut the hair underneath the mushroom at the sideburns.

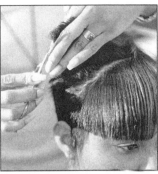

Step 6•To make sure your cut is even, lift ribbons around the head at the crown level and trim where necessary.

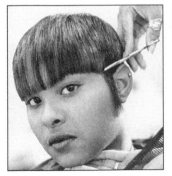

Step 7•Trim the ends of the hair at the sideburns at an angle toward the face. The sideburns should end just above the bottom of the ear-lobes.

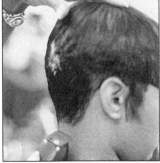

Step 8•Trim the neckline with light strokes of the electric clipper. Comb and style. Curls can be added to the crown for a whole new look.

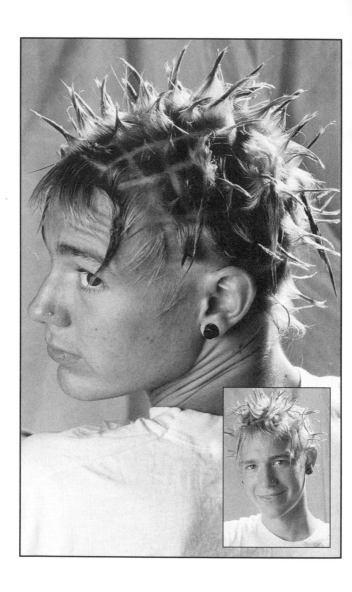

Spike

Wilder than wild, this variation on the standard razor cut experiments with using the clipper's edge to cut a pattern of squares and rectangles into the hair. The tuft of hair in each section is twisted into a spike. This post-punk ragamuffin look lets it all hang out—or rather stand straight up—with the help of a touch of gel. Wear this one at an upcoming concert and there'll be more than one star attraction.

⏰ 60 minutes

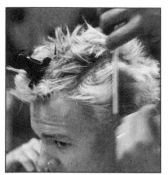

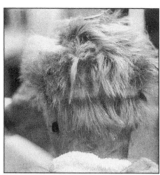

Step 1•Cut the hair dry. Section off the crown of the hair with a clip.

Step 2•Bulk cut the rest of the hair to about 4 inches all over.

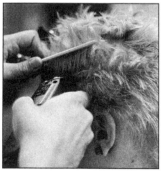

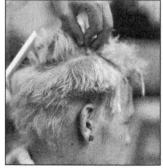

Step 3•Using an electric clipper, cut a horizontal line into the hair just below the crown. This will be the first line in what will be a checkerboard pattern. Each piece of hair in the checkerboard will be about 1 square inch in size.

Step 4•Using the edge of the bare clipper, cut a wide line about 3 inches above the nape of the neck from ear to ear. Cut a second line 3 inches above the first.

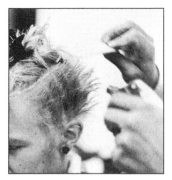

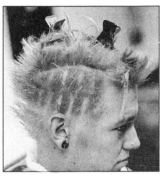

Step 5 • Cut narrow vertical lines to connect the horizontal lines you created at the crown and at the midpoint at the back of the head.

Note vertical and horizontal lines in this side view.

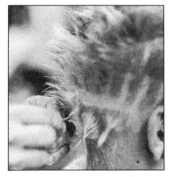

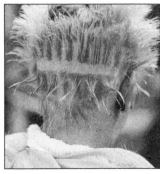

Step 6 • Begin twisting the hair in each rectangle. Add a bit of gel so that these spikes will hold.

Back view showing checkerboard pattern and spikes.

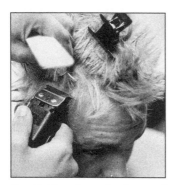

Step 7•Move forward to the top of the head, and remove the clip at the crown. Leave hair at forehead for bangs.

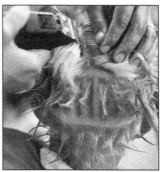

Step 8•In the remaining hair at the crown make vertical lines from the crown to the hairline.

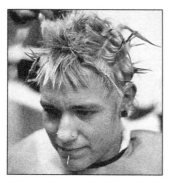

Now you've completed the checkerboard pattern.

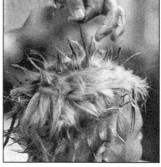

Step 9•Apply gel to fingers and twist the hair of each section individually.

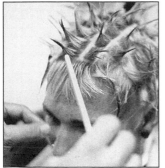
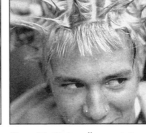

Step 10•Comb bangs forward. Establish 3 inch guidelines for the bang cut.

Step 11•Twist all remaining sections.

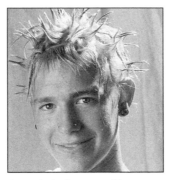

Step 12•A glorious, wilder you.

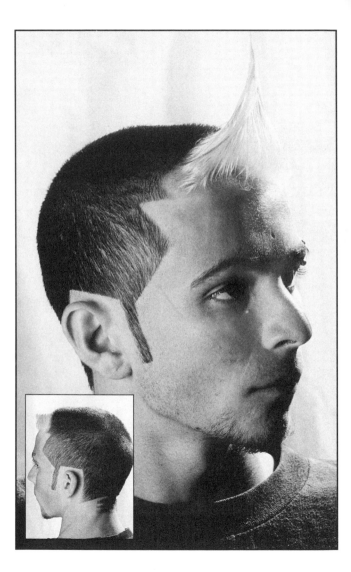

Rooster's Crown

Strut your stuff. Wear the Rooster's Crown. Neat yet daring, the hair is cut very short on the top and sides. A razor cut accents the nape of the neck. The hairline and sideburns are shaped precisely to show off the crown—a bleached bang that can peak or flow, depending on the rooster's crow.

🕐 45 minutes

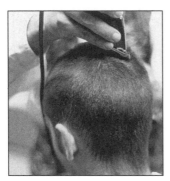

Step 1•Cut dry hair evenly, about ¾ inch all over. Leave 4-inch bangs that have been bleached for 45 minutes (see bleaching directions on page 28).

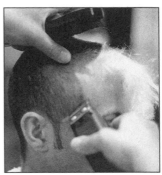

Step 2•Use electric clippers to sculpt and shape the hairline around the face.

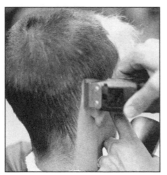

Step 3•Create a dramatic clean angle at the sides.

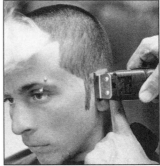

Step 4•Define the sideburns.

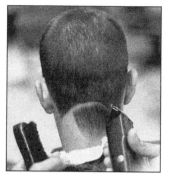

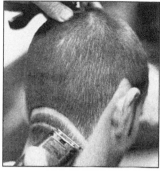

Step 5•Shape the neckline in a wide wedge. Razor cut a gentle sloping line.

Step 6•Create a second line about ½ inch below the first line.

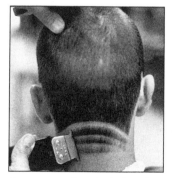

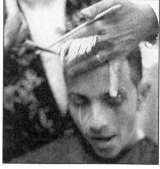

Step 7•Complete the look with a third line.

Step 8•Trim the bangs, apply gel, and style. Experiment with different twists and colors, or sweep the bangs over the eye.

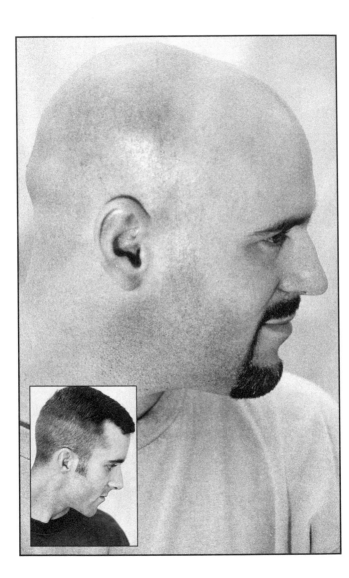

Ultimate

Take it all off and parade your beautiful head. Arthur carefully shaves his head nearly every day with shaving gel and a razor. Bald is beautiful!

To shave off your hair, section it and use bare electric clippers to shear it from back to front.

If you can't go all the way, choose a Fade (as shown in the inset picture). Cut the Fade short on top and nearly bare, about $\frac{1}{8}$ inch at the sides and back. It's the step before the Ultimate.

🕓 25 minutes

ROUGHING IT

Roughing it

You're looking beyond good in your Rough Cut. Heads turn as you walk down the street. Not only have you become an expert cutter and stylist, you've now begun to experiment with far-out variations.

Here are some ways to use color, curls, and styling products to enhance your terrific Rough Cuts.

- Add dreadlocks to Spike and Tango.
- Dye the mane of Soho/The Village purple.
- Bleach the length of hair at the back of Petals.
- Curl the bangs of Spun Sugar.
- Use gel to twist a few fun spikes in Flipped Script.

Experiment with your Rough Cut, and before you know it, your little sister will shave off all her hair! Everybody loves Rough Cuts and having fun with hairstyles.

They're the ultimate.

STEP-BY-STEP GUIDES FOR HAIR, NAILS, AND ACCESSORIES

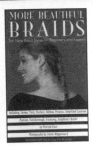

BEAUTIFUL BRAIDS
and
MORE BEAUTIFUL BRAIDS

The Step-by-Step Guides to Braiding Styles

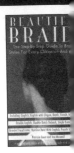

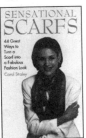

SENSATIONAL SCARFS

Create Fantastic
New Looks for
Your Wardrobe

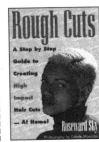

ROUGH CUTS

Create Fantas
High-Impact
Hair Cuts at H

CROWN PUBLISHERS, INC.
400 Hahn Road, Westminster, MD 21157
Attn: CTP Order Entry
010-05

Please send me:
❑ *Beautiful Braids* ❑ *More Beautiful Braids*
❑ *Sensational Scarfs* ❑ *Rough Cuts* ❑ *Hot Tips*

I enclose my check or money order for $5.99 (per book) plus
$1.50 postage and handling charge (per book). If I wish, I
may return the book postpaid within ten days for full refund.

Name _____

Address _____

City _____ State _____ Zip _____

Please add sales tax where applicable.

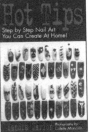

HOT TIPS

Create Incredib
Professional N
at Home

Crown Trade Pap